D0614362

BARBARA PEARLMAN'S
4–Week Stomach & Waist Shape-up

Also by Barbara Pearlman

BARBARA PEARLMAN'S DANCE EXERCISES

BARBARA PEARLMAN'S SLENDERCISES

BARBARA PEARLMAN'S
4–Week Stomach & Waist Shape-up

Barbara Pearlman
Photographs by George Bennett

A DOLPHIN BOOK
DOUBLEDAY & COMPANY, INC.
GARDEN CITY, NEW YORK
1983

Library of Congress Cataloging in Publication Data

Pearlman, Barbara.
    Barbara Pearlman's 4–week stomach & waist shape-up.

"A Dolphin book."
    1. Reducing exercises.   2. Exercise for
women.   3. Abdomen.   I. Title.   II. Title:
4–week stomach & waist shape-up.   III. Title:
4–week stomach & waist shape-up.   IV. Title:
4–week stomach & waist shape-up.
RA781.6.P397   1983   646.7′5
ISBN: 0-385-18353-4
Library of Congress Catalog Card Number: 82–45520

Copyright © 1983 by Barbara Pearlman

ALL RIGHTS RESERVED
PRINTED IN THE UNITED STATES OF AMERICA
FIRST EDITION

To Miriam

Grateful appreciation to those who have lent their expertise—Lindy Hess, Laura Van Wormer, Alex Gotfryd, George Bennett, Lynn Padwe and Richard Ohanesian. My gratitude to Capezio Ballet Makers for their contribution to this book.

A very special thanks to my husband, Stephen, and my son, Aaron, for their loving support.

Contents

Introduction

If zipping everything up isn't a zip, and you take pride of ownership in your body, your work is set out for you in this waist-slimming, tummy-trimming shape-up plan. The exercises in this program are specifically designed to tone and firm your waist and abdominals, two problem zones where muscles tend to slacken and excess fat tends to accumulate. By regularly practicing this collection of thirty-two toners, you'll begin to see a visible difference in your midsection in just a month's time. And if you're willing to devote more than twenty minutes a day to your practice sessions, and pour on a bit of extra steam, results might be evident even sooner.

In addition to trimming and slimming your waist and abdominals, the exercises will help you become more flexible and supple. They will heighten your ability to move with grace, agility, and ease. In just a short time, it will be possible to place greater demands on your body, not only while you exercise, but throughout the day, in everything you do. And although the waist and abdominals are the prime figure targets for this program, other problem spots will derive a "bonus" toning as well.

The exercises in this program will smooth away bulges, trim off inches and change flabbiness to firmly controlled curves. In short, they will recontour your midsection. But they won't dissolve excess pounds. This is the time to launch a diet, either on your own or possibly with the guidance of a physician, if your problem is due partially to overweight. Find a realistic pounds-off plan and be prepared to stick to it. This is essential because the longer your stomach remains expanded due to excess weight, the greater the chance the abdominal wall will lose its shape.

Dieting is never the sole solution. It won't guarantee you the figure you hope to attain. Unless your abdominals are strong and firm, your stomach will continue to protrude, even if your weight is right on target. Exercise affects the shape of your body; diet affects its weight. Neither can do the job of the other. Combine the two, however, and the dual line of attack can work wonders. At the conclusion of each week's exercise segment, you'll find some no-nonsense tips for figure control and weight loss. If you are intent and serious about taking off some weight, try to keep these hints in mind. They're sensible, easy-to-follow, and best of all, they really work.

Ideally, your waistline should be slim, flexible, and, above all, unencumbered by rolls of superfluous flesh. By following this program, you will attain more of an hourglass shape, not necessarily à la Scarlett O'Hara, but suited to your individual proportions and bone structure. (You can't whittle your waist to 23″ when it's structurally 27″ at its flattest.) Each woman is uniquely built and should work toward achieving *her* best proportions within the realm of her own bone structure and figure type. Devote your energies to getting your body into its own state of perfection, without comparing it to others. We need not aspire to all look alike. What is important is that we all look our best.

Whereas a bit of "excess" *might* be alluring and provocative on your buttocks and hips, around your middle it just is not. By tapering your waist and firming your tummy, you will look and feel sexier as well. When you're flabby, out of shape, and feel unattractive, you convey this self-image to your partner. On the other hand, if you look in the mirror and like what you see, you will respond accordingly while making love. When you're proud of your body and you know it's the best it can be, you're naturally more receptive to having others look at you and touch you as well.

Poor posture can truly play havoc with your figure as well as with your body. When you slouch, your abdominals not only sag and protrude, but your waistline becomes obscured as well. By allowing your upper body to slip downward, you not only destroy the line of your waist, but you place an increased burden on your entire lower body, in particular your back. Unfortunately, many women simply do not know and cannot feel what good posture is. It certainly isn't a military-like shoulders-back-chest-out stance that you probably learned in grade school.

In order to envision proper standing posture, think of your body as a series of pearls strung one under the other on a single string. If the string is slack, all the pearls fall out of line. Correct standing posture consists of keeping your head lifted, your chin tucked in, and your pelvis tilted slightly forward. With your head and chin in their proper position, the curve in your cervical spine will flatten. By contracting your buttock muscles and tilting your pelvis forward, the curve of your lumbar spine flattens. Remember, however, posture embraces all positions of the body and is equally crucial when you're sitting or lying down. Once you develop strength in the muscles that hold you erect, you will attain a more graceful, youthful appearance. Not only will you look better and deceptively slender, but your body will function better as well.

In the lifelong contest between you and your back, there's absolutely no substitute for good posture and muscle tone. By abusing the back (holding it out of line) or neglecting it (depriving it of exercise), the muscles that support the spine lose their elasticity and strength. The result—aches, pains, and overall body fatigue. As you practice the exercises in this program, constantly remind yourself to pull in your abdominals. When lying flat, press your spine against the floor in order to keep your back from arching unnecessarily. Remember, too, the effect of these exercises is cumulative. The success of strengthening your abdominals (and, in turn, your back) depends on you and how willing you are to perform these exercises regularly.

This four-week exercise plan can also serve as a super after-pregnancy shape-up. During the nine months of pregnancy, the abdominal muscles and tissues stretch to accommodate a uterus that will expand to about twenty times its usual size. Naturally, in the process, the waist thickens considerably. Once your physician gives you the green light to exercise, begin with Week I and proceed at your own pace. Take all the time you need. Don't feel compelled to complete each segment in a week's time or to follow the suggested repetitions. As you regain muscular strength and control, the movements will become consistently easier for you to do. Once your tone, stamina, and pre-pregnancy shape have returned, you can use all the exercises as an effective maintenance regime.

There's a simple abdominal exercise that can be done just about anytime and anywhere and nobody will even know you're exercising. You can practice this inconspicuous exercise when you're at your desk, soaking in a tub, or waiting on the grocery check-out line. Pull in your abdominal muscles as tight as possible, but don't hold your breath. Maintain the contraction for six slow counts, then relax. As you become more adept at this exercise, you will be able to hold the contraction longer and longer. I try to punctuate my day with this simple drill, be it while I'm reading, cooking, or applying my makeup. You'll find the more frequently you practice the abdominal contraction, the easier and more natural it will become.

In general, try to make it a point to "steal" an extra stretch, twist, or bend whenever and wherever you can. "Sneaky Exercises" (those that you can do more or less invisibly) are a constructive way to use time. They also take the boredom out of enforced "waits." While you water your overhead hanging plants, or dust a high shelf, reach a tiny bit more than necessary. Or resist climbing your kitchen step stool and attempt to stretch for the canned goods instead. While doing household chores, try to exaggerate your movements in order to activate your muscles and stimulate the circulation in your waist and abdominal areas. All these subtle, extra motions can help you redesign your body. In addition, they keep you supple and flexible.

In the morning, before I get out of bed, I spend a minute or two awakening my body with a head to toe, total stretch. Lie fully extended on your back, arms relaxed at your sides. Flex your right foot by pressing your heel down. At the same time, stretch your right arm overhead, palm up. The left side of your body should remain perfectly relaxed. Release the arm and foot and repeat the stretch on the left side. Try not to arch your back unnecessarily as you stretch. This exercise really works wonders for activating the circulation and "dekinking" the body after a night's sleep.

The movements in this program are based on a blend of techniques: dance exercise warm-ups, modified yoga postures, orthopedic exercises, and a short running in place segment to stimulate your cardiorespiratory system. I do not want to suggest, however, that this program is the answer to all your fitness needs. It is, instead, a plan designed to focus on two problem zones—the waist and the abdominals. Ideally, you should supplement a toning, stretch program of this sort with a regular aerobic activity that appeals to you. Aerobic exercises are those that commit you to consume more oxygen. Any sport, game, or rhythmic movement that you continue for *at least* twenty minutes without stopping for rest qualifies as aerobic activity.

The running in place segment (you may substitute jumping rope) should be done *after* you complete the eight exercises in the sequence. If you wish to extend this portion of your sessions to more than three minutes, by all means do so. Wear a pair of sneakers or running shoes. Appropriate footwear is necessary to cushion your steps and lessen the chance of injury. A padded or carpeted surface is also suggested. You can run with your arms relaxed at your sides, or if you prefer, raise your arms overhead for an extra stretch in your waistline. Ideally, you should try to pace yourself at about sixty steps per minute. But never strain. If you find sixty too many at first, start with less and gradually work toward your goal. One way to determine if you're running at the right pace is to carry on a conversation while you move. If you find it a strain to speak, slow down somewhat. After you run, be sure to cool down by walking around. Take big strides and continue until your breathing has returned to normal.

In order to exercise successfully with this plan, try to work for approximately twenty minutes a day for an entire month. Follow the program according to its design. As the weeks progress, the exercises gradually become more difficult. This should pose no problem. By following the order in which I've placed the movements, you will be sufficiently prepared to assume greater demands on your body. If, however, you find an exercise too difficult, never push or strain. Take the signals from your body and let up a bit. YOU NEED NOT AGONIZE TO EXERCISE! Don't become discouraged if you can't immediately assume the positions as shown in the photographs. They are presented as goals to be worked toward rather than what should be copied immediately. If you're patient and persevere, your capabilities will expand and improve each day. Should you find the number of repetitions called for excessive, decrease them according to your stamina and ability. In fact, if you're really out of shape, you may want to devote more than one week to each segment. Don't be too severe on yourself if you happen to miss or skip a day. Simply resume where you left off and forge on!

With each exercise, discover the breathing pattern that gives the movement maximum support. This is important in order to keep your muscles well oxygenated. Oftentimes, especially if you are a beginner, the tendency is to hold your breath or to breathe in a shallow manner. This robs you of energy. When you're first learning an exercise, relax and just breathe as naturally as possible. Then, once you're familiar with the movement, pay close attention to proper breath control. Usually, any lifted movement, when accompanied by an inhalation of breath will become fuller and more enriched. Try to breathe in through your nose and out through your mouth. Exhale as though you are blowing out a candle. Generally, you will use your abdominals during the exhalation and relax them during the inhalation. Learn to control your breathing so that you can use it to your advantage.

As you perform the various exercises in this program, remember to separate your torso from your hips by maintaining a "lift" in your upper body. This will help you derive a more complete stretch from each exercise, and it will also serve to rev up the circulation in the waist and abdominal areas. You will also experience a greater pull on your waist when doing exercises such as the one on page 50 if you keep the palm of the upper arm facing the ceiling. By positioning the hand in this way, you are assured a full stretch, all the way down to your hips.

You're probably working too rapidly if you complete the

daily program in far less than twenty minutes time. Slow down somewhat. Never sacrifice speed for thoroughness. Should you wish to devote more than twenty minutes to your daily practice sessions, you may increase the number of repetitions, repeat several of the exercises in the segment or you may include exercises from previous weeks. You can also increase the running segment, working up to a possible ten or even fifteen minutes. Once you've completed the four-week plan, it can be repeated again and again, or you can combine the thirty-two exercises in an endless variety of personally designed routines. Completion of this program will, hopefully, create enough of an exercise spirit that you will continue long after the four weeks are up.

No area betrays a woman's age faster than her "middle." As soon as it is streamlined, and properly proportioned, her entire body appears more beautiful. Now I'm not implying it's a cinch to whittle your waistline or tone your tummy. It takes considerable effort, commitment, and above all, the desire for results. But it can be done! I've designed an easy-to-follow, effective program that requires no special equipment or expensive exercise gadgets. And best of all, it can be done right at home. Stick with the program for an entire month, and you'll not only look slimmer and firmer through your middle, but your entire figure will look lovelier as well. Have fun with it. Good luck and happy stretching.

Barbara Pearlman

BARBARA PEARLMAN'S
4–Week Stomach & Waist Shape-up

Some Helpful Hints

- Consult a physician before beginning this program if you've had a recent illness or injury or have a special or chronic physical condition.

- Establish the "Exercise Habit." Exercise at the same time each day, if possible. This insures you won't forget. Find a time that appeals to your own body clock. Preferences are really quite personal and *when* is not nearly as crucial as *whether*. Avoid exercising right after a heavy meal (it inhibits digestion) or right before bedtime (it's too stimulating).

- It's much more fun to exercise to music. Music not only helps you execute the movements with greater rhythm and grace, but it adds to the overall enjoyment of your practice time. Choose music that appeals to you and change it according to your mood each day.

- *Do not exercise on a bare floor.* A carpeted or padded surface that cushions your spine is essential. You should consider investing in an exercise mat or make one yourself. (See instructions on page 3.)

- Your practice space (approximately eight square feet) should be clean, clear of obstructions, and free of drafts. Cold air, be it from a window, fan, or air-conditioner, hitting warm muscles can cause cramps or spasms.

- Wear clothing that allows for maximum freedom of movement. Tights and leotards are ideal in that they are designed for movement and keep your muscles warm as well.

- Avoid stopping and starting once you've begun to exercise. Interruptions are not only time consuming, but they cause a loss of momentum and continuity. Insure as much privacy and quiet as possible.

- Concentrate as you move in order to give total attention to correct alignment and technique. Focus on the stretching process as it affects the various parts of your body.

- Work in front of a full-length mirror if possible. Let your eyes assist you in making corrections and adjustments.

- At the beginning of each week, in order to perform the exercises properly, I suggest you do the following: Place the book where you can refer to it easily. Look at the photos in order to get the general impression of the exercise. Next, read the accompanying instructions just as you would a recipe in which each ingredient must be noted. Then reread the exercise as you slowly pace through it. Naturally, the first day of each week might take a bit more time in that you will be learning the eight exercises for the first time.

How to Make Your Own Exercise Mat

You can whip up your own exercise mat with relatively little time, money, and effort. All you need for this project are two large beach towels of identical size and a foam rubber pad, which is available in various thicknesses at most sewing centers or department stores. The pad should be about one inch narrower and two inches shorter than the dimensions of the towels. Stitch the sides and one end of the towels together (use a sewing machine if one's available). Turn the towels inside out and insert the pad. Close the other end of the towels with snap fasteners (for easy laundering). That's all there is to it. . . . You have your personal exercise mat.

Week I
Introduction

You're off and on your way to a slimmer, trimmer figure. Take it easy, take it slow. Never push yourself in order to assume an extreme position. With practice, your muscles will begin to obey your commands. If you haven't exercised for a long time, don't be alarmed if at first you experience a bit of muscular soreness. It's only natural and should be expected. Simply continue with more of the same movements. A soak in a warm tub can also ease minor aches and stiffness.

Remember too, the same exercise can feel quite different from one day to the next. That's because your body changes constantly and reacts from day to day to many variables—the weather, your moods, the amount of sleep you had, etc. One day you might feel in fighting form, the next, not nearly as refreshed.

1. Cat Stretch

Placement: Begin on your hands and knees, hands shoulder-width apart. Keep your back straight.

Movement: Round your back, lower your head, and contract your abdominals. Hold for five slow counts, then return to the straight-back position.

Repetition: Repeat eight times.

As you contract, exhale through your mouth. Inhale through your nose as you return to the original position.

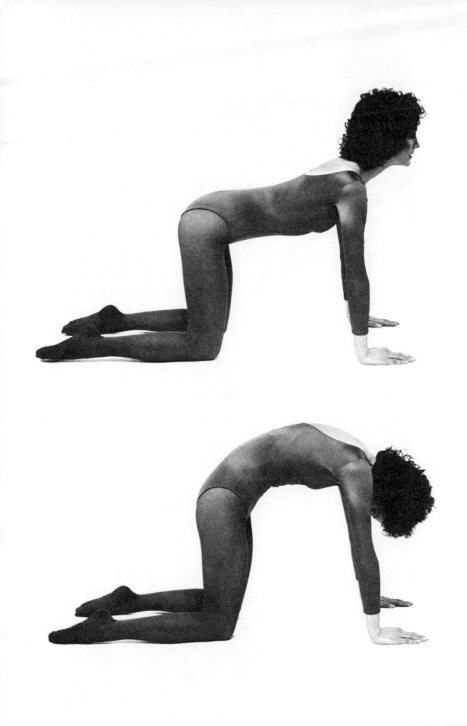

2. Side Slide

Placement: Sit tailor fashion, ankles crossed, back erect. Rest your hands on the floor near your knees.

Movement: Lean your upper body to the left as you slide your left hand on the floor away from your body. Arch your right arm overhead, palm up. Bounce up and down four times. Return to the original position and repeat to the right. Repeat six times to each side, then rest for six slow counts.

Repetition: Repeat total sequence two times.

Keep your buttocks stationary as you stretch to the side. This exercise should be performed slowly and rhythmically.

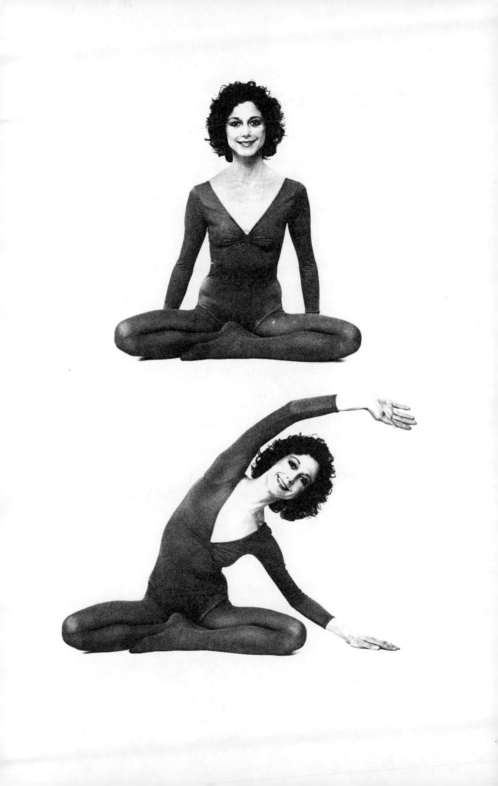

3. Rowboat

Placement: Sit with your knees slightly bent. Place the soles of your feet wide apart on the floor. Extend your arms in front at chest level, palms down.

Movement: Stretch your upper body forward from your hips as you lower your head between your knees. Slide your hands on the floor in front of your head. Next, release back and straighten your legs until the small of your back touches the floor, toes pointed. Repeat the complete forward and back motion eight times. Rest six counts, then repeat.

Repetition: Repeat the total sequence three times.

As you release back, contract your abdominal and buttock muscles in order to maintain balance and control. Inhale on the forward motion, exhale on the release back.

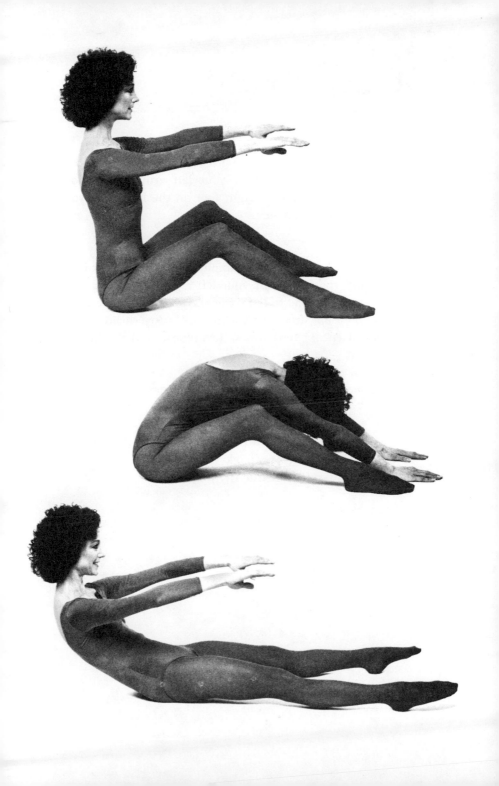

4. Leg Touch

Placement: Lie on your back with your left leg extended in front, toes pointed. Rest your left arm on the floor overhead. Place your right foot on the floor and your right arm at your side.

Movement: Contract your abdominals and press your back against the floor. Lift your left arm and left leg, trying to touch one to the other. Lower both to the original position, stretching the arm as far overhead as possible. Repeat twelve times, then repeat on the right side.

Repetition: Repeat total sequence two times.

Keep your abdominals contracted throughout this exercise in order to prevent your back from arching. Work at a moderate tempo and breathe rhythmically.

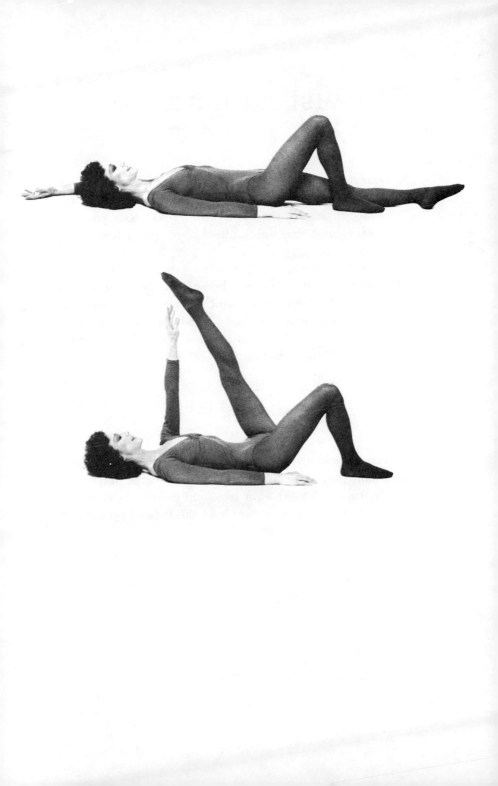

5. Twist Around

Placement: Sit with your left knee bent and resting on the floor. Cross your right foot over your left thigh and place it close to the thigh on the floor. Rest your left heel against your right buttock, arms relaxed.

Movement: Twist your upper body from the waist to your left. Place your right hand on your right heel and your left palm on the floor behind you. Look over your left shoulder. Hold this position for a slow count of twenty. Repeat the twist to your right.

Repetition: Two times to each side.

As you remain in the twisted position, keep your torso lifted and your abdominals contracted. Breathe deeply and evenly. Inhale through your nose and exhale through your mouth. If you wish, you may hold the twisted position for longer than twenty counts.

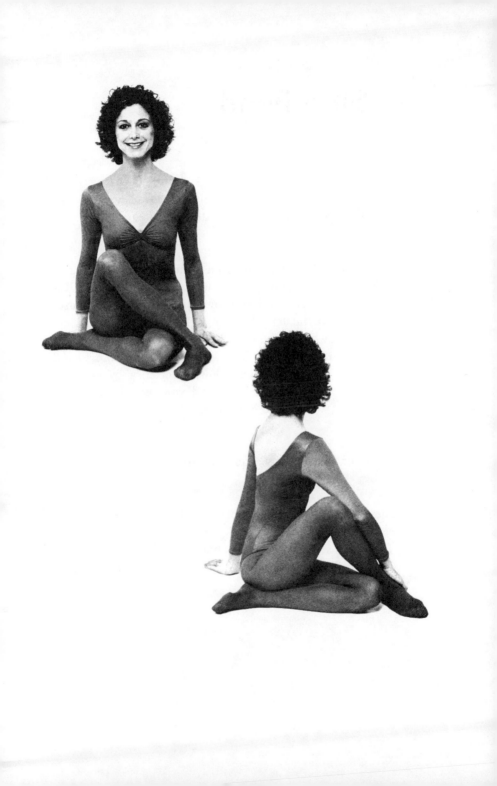

6. Side Bend

Placement: Sit tall with your legs extended to the sides, toes pointed, legs turned out. Interlace your hands behind your head, elbows wide apart.

Movement: Bend sideways from your waist to the right. Lower your elbow as close to the leg as possible. Return to center position, lifting high through the torso. Repeat to the left. Repeat eight times to each side. Next, lower your head, bring your elbows together and bounce up and down eight times as close to the floor as possible. Uncurl slowly, vertebra by vertebra until your back is straight and your elbows are wide apart.

Repetition: Repeat total sequence three times.

Remember to keep your elbows wide apart on the side stretch. Don't be concerned if you cannot extend your legs as far apart as shown in the photograph. Work gradually toward a fuller stretch. Lift your torso high each time you return to the center position.

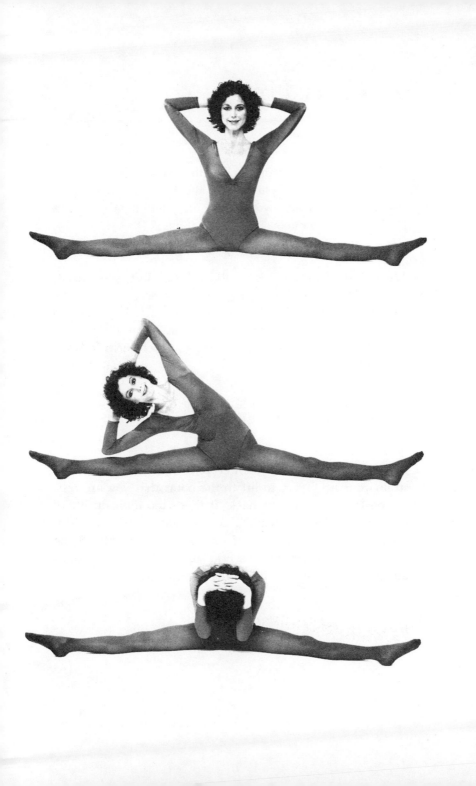

7. Curl Up

Placement: Lie on your back with your knees bent, feet wide apart and parallel on the floor. Interlace your fingers and rest your head in your hands, elbows touching the floor.

Movement: Contract your abdominals. Lift your head, neck, shoulders, upper back, and middle back off the floor as you bring your elbows together. Roll back to the floor slowly, elbows touching last. Repeat six times. Draw your knees to your chest and rock them forward and back six times.

Repetition: Repeat total sequence three times.

As you roll off the floor, lower your chin in order not to strain your neck. Try to lift to the point that you are resting on the small of your back. If that's too difficult, lift to your middle back instead. Take a breath before you lift, then exhale as you roll up. If you are unable to lift off the floor, tuck your feet under a firm support that will serve as an anchor. This will facilitate the movement.

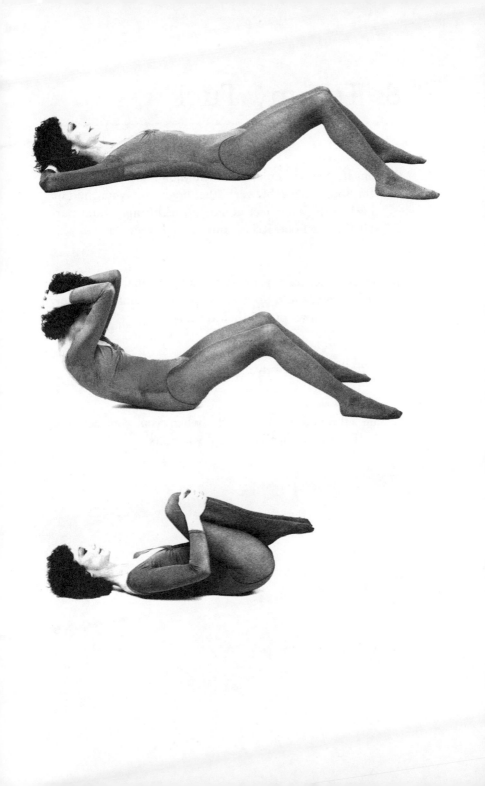

8. Tummy Tuck

Placement: Lie on your back with your knees bent. Allow for some space between the floor and your middle back. Place your feet about hip-width apart and parallel on the floor. Relax your arms at your sides.

Movement: Contract your abdominals so that your stomach tightens and your spine presses against the floor. Hold six slow counts, then relax.

Repetition: Repeat twelve times.

Exhale (through your mouth) when you contract and inhale (through your nose) when you relax.

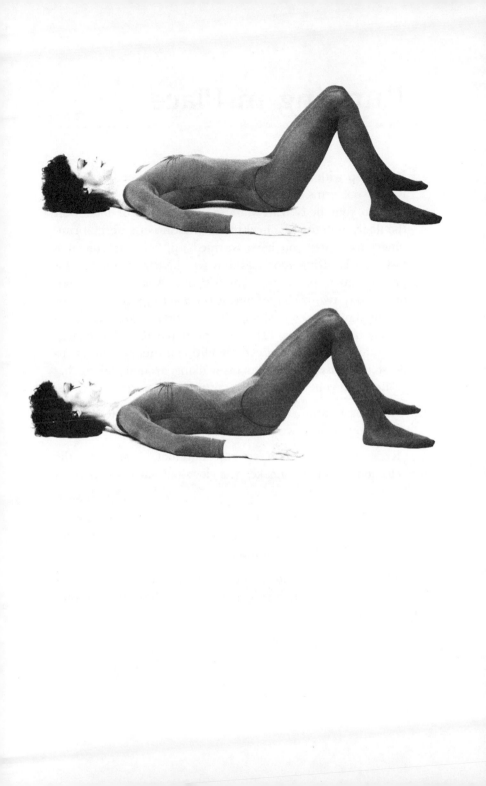

Running in Place

Warm up with a slow jog for the first thirty or forty steps. Relax your arms or bend them at the elbows, holding them close to your body. Lift your feet three or four inches off the floor, imitating the heel-toe alternation of a normal running pace. After you have warmed up, begin to run at a faster pace, lifting your legs and feet higher. Maintain this pace for about one minute the first day. Add a second minute on day two or three, and a third on day four, five, or six. By day seven, you should be comfortable with approximately three minutes. (If you're prepared for a longer segment, and you wish to devote additional time, by all means do so.) *Always* cool down by walking around, taking big strides until your breathing has returned to normal.

- Running to music is the best way to keep up a steady beat and to enjoy it as well.

- Resist the temptation to run barefoot. You need the cushioning of a sneaker or jogging shoe to prevent soreness.

- In order to "earn points," you should raise each foot a minimum of eight inches off the floor and achieve a minimum of sixty steps a minute.

- To estimate your rate of steps per minute, for fifteen seconds count each time your left foot hits the floor and multiply by four.

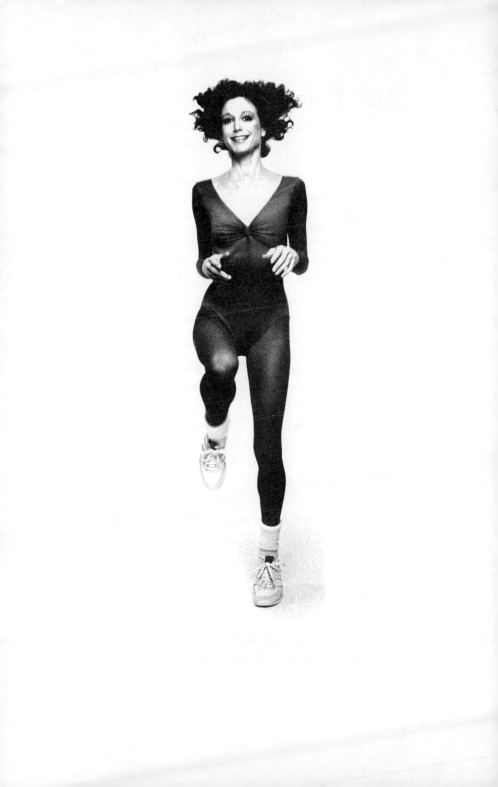

Big Loser Tips

- Timing can be just as important as motivation. Set yourself up for diet success. Be certain you're ready to make losing weight a top priority.

- Think thin! Banish your "fat" clothes such as baggy pants and shapeless tops. If you keep a "fat wardrobe" waiting in the closet, just in case, you're setting yourself up for failure.

- Take one day at a time and set *realistic* goals.

- Don't weigh yourself every day. Once a week is enough.

- Avoid crash or blitz diets that restrict food intake to near starvation. Sure, you might lose weight, but you'll only gain it back twice as quickly.

- Try keeping a food diary for a week. Record *everything* you eat each day. This is one way to find out whether or not you've been inadvertently consuming more than you should. Note what you eat, when you eat, and your mood at the time.

- Heighten your eating awareness. Put everything you eat on a plate and use utensils when appropriate. This forces you to maintain eye contact with your food and also helps heighten your awareness of how much you are eating.

- At parties or get-togethers, don't stand near the hors d'oeuvres or sit next to the "nibbles." It's too tempting.

- Don't eat on the run or while standing in the kitchen. Sit at a table, eat slowly, and savor each and every bite.

Week II
Introduction

~~~~~~

The eight exercises in this week's segment are somewhat tougher than those you worked on last week. But don't be concerned, you're prepared to tackle them! With daily practice and repetition, you'll find they will become consistently easier to do. As you improve, you will experience a wonderful feeling of accomplishment. Give yourself an occasional pat on the back and be proud of your progress. You deserve it.

1. Torso Lift

Placement: Lie on your right side. Use your right elbow to support your torso which should be slightly raised. Place your left hand on the floor in front of your body for additional support. Extend your left leg behind as high as possible, knee down, toes pointed.

Movement: Bend your knee to your chest as you lower your head. Try to touch one to the other. Next, lift your body and head as you thrust the leg back to the original position. Repeat ten times. Repeat with the right leg.

Repetition: Repeat two times on each side.

As you bend your knee toward your chest, contract your abdominals and exhale. Inhale on the lifting motion.

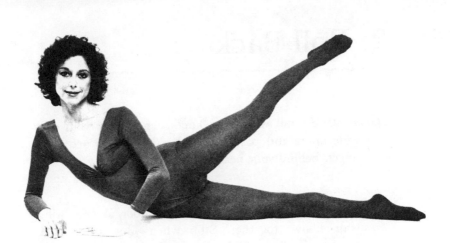

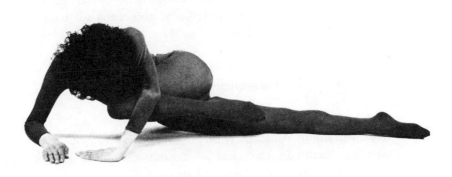

2. Roll Back

Placement: Sit tall with your knees bent. Place your feet wide apart and parallel on the floor. Interlace your fingers behind your head, elbows wide apart.

Movement: Roll halfway back to the floor as you bring your elbows together. Stop when your lower back touches the floor. Hold four slow counts, then lift to the original position, elbows wide apart. Repeat slowly six times. Next, relax your abdominals by straightening your legs, round your back, and reach for your toes. Bounce up and down six times.

Repetition: Repeat the sequence three times.

Make certain to contract your abdominals when you roll back and maintain the "hold" at your maximum stress point. Exhale on the roll back, inhale on the lift.

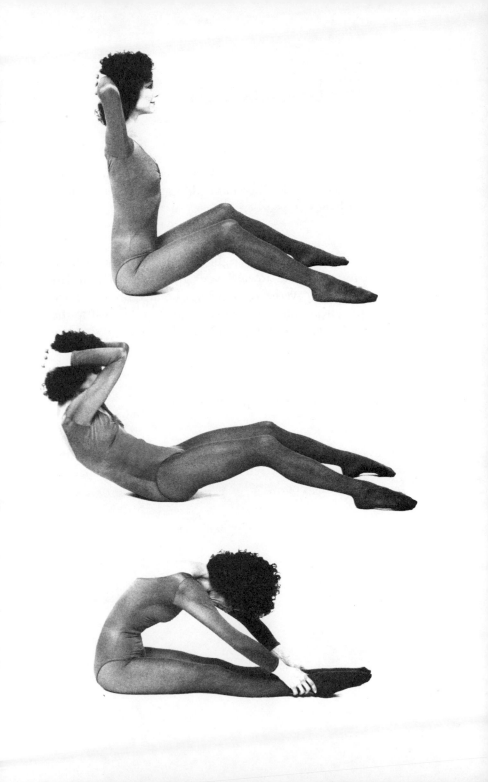

3. Side Stretch

Placement: Sit tall with your legs extended as far to the sides as possible, toes pointed, legs turned out. Rest your hands on your legs.

Movement: Lean to your right from your waist. Stretch your right hand toward your right foot as your left arm arches overhead, palm up. Bounce up and down four times. Return to center position and repeat to the left. Repeat six times to each side. Rest for six slow counts.

Repetition: Repeat the sequence two times.

Always return to a lifted center position before stretching to either side. As you stretch to one side, press the opposite buttock into the floor.

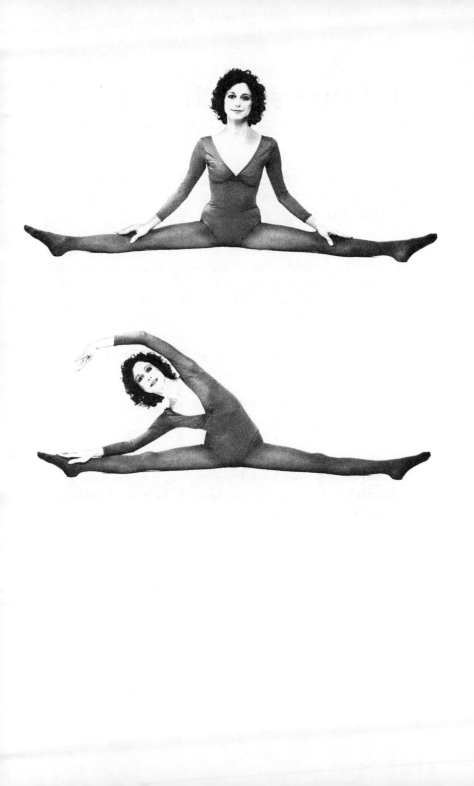

4. Superstretch

Placement: Lie on your back with your knees drawn close to your chest. Place your hands just below (not on) your knees.

Movement: Extend your right leg forward until it is straight and practically touching the floor. At the same time, stretch your right arm on the floor overhead. Bring the arm and leg back into position and repeat on the left side. Repeat four times on each side. Hug your knees to your chest and hold for four slow counts.

Repetition: Repeat the sequence four times.

In order to keep your back from arching, contract your abdominals on the arm/leg extension. Exhale on the extension, inhale on the release.

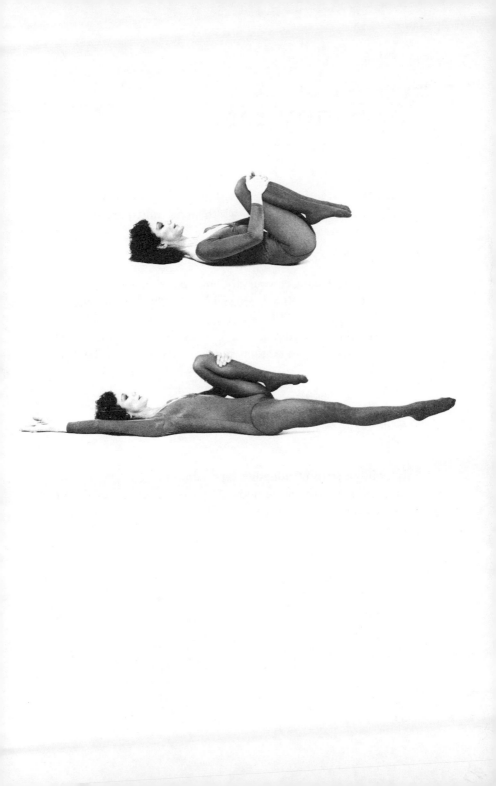

5. Fanny Lift

Placement: Lie on your back, knees bent. Place your feet on the floor about hip-width apart and parallel. Rest your arms at your sides.

Movement: Contract your abdominals. Peel your back off the floor vertebra by vertebra. At the height of your lift, there should be a straight diagonal line from your shoulders to your knees. Try not to arch your back. Hold four counts, then slowly roll your spine back to the floor.

Repetition: Repeat twelve times.

Imagine a strip of adhesive tape running down your back and another strip on the floor. As you roll down, match one to the other. Take four counts to lift, four to hold, and four to release.

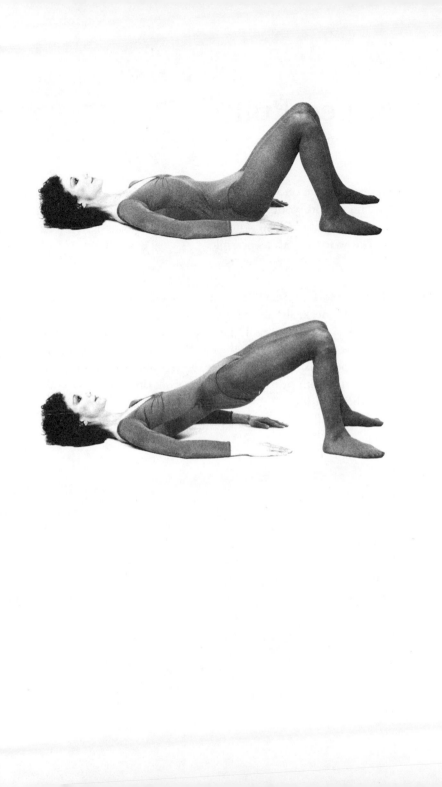

6. Leg Pull

Placement: Lie on your back. Extend your right leg on the floor and your left leg upward, toes pointed, foot turned out. Clasp your hands around your left leg as close to the calf as possible.

Movement: Contract your abdominals. Slowly lift your head, neck, shoulders, and upper back off the floor. At the same time, pull the leg toward you. Hold three slow counts, then roll your body back to the floor. Repeat six times. Lower your leg and roll your head gently from side to side a total of six times. Repeat with the right leg.

Repetition: Repeat the sequence two times.

If you are unable to clasp your hands on your calf, place them further up your leg instead. You may also bend the forward extended leg should you find extending it on the floor too difficult. Make certain to include the head roll motion. It serves to relax the muscles in the neck and is important as a "punctuation" movement.

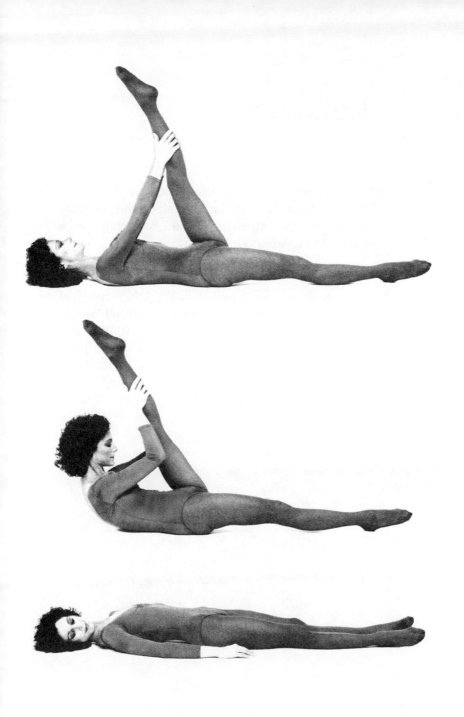

7. Rollover

Placement: Lie on your back, left leg extended in front. Rest your right foot on the left thigh, knee pointing up. Extend your arms on the floor, slightly below shoulder level, palms down.

Movement: Roll your knee as far to the left as possible. Bounce it up and down eight times. Then roll back to the original position. Repeat four times. Repeat with the left knee.

Repetition: Repeat the sequence two times.

Try to keep your shoulders stationary and your hands in place. Keep your abdominals contracted and your head relaxed.

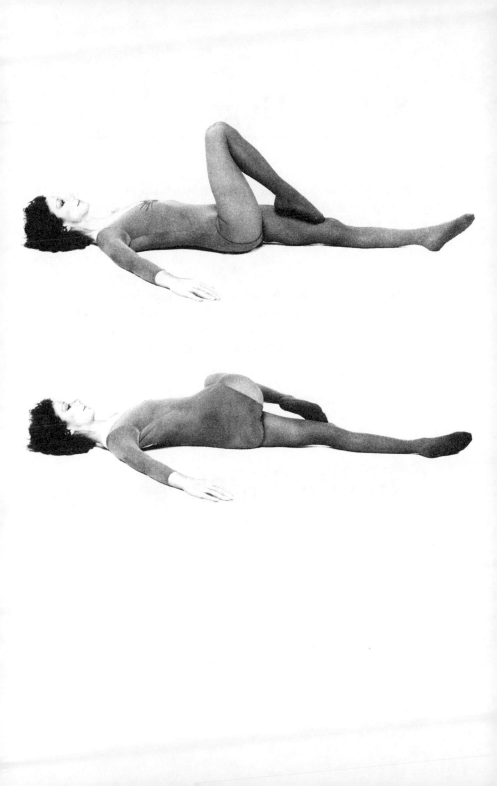

8. Knee Hug

Placement: Sit with your right leg extended in front, foot pointed and turned out. Bend the left leg and rest the foot against the right thigh. Raise your arms overhead, back erect.

Movement: Reach forward from your hips, lowering your torso over your right leg. Lift to the original position, pulling up through your waist. Repeat twelve times. Repeat with the left leg extended in front.

Repetition: Repeat two times with each leg.

Running in Place

(Three minutes)

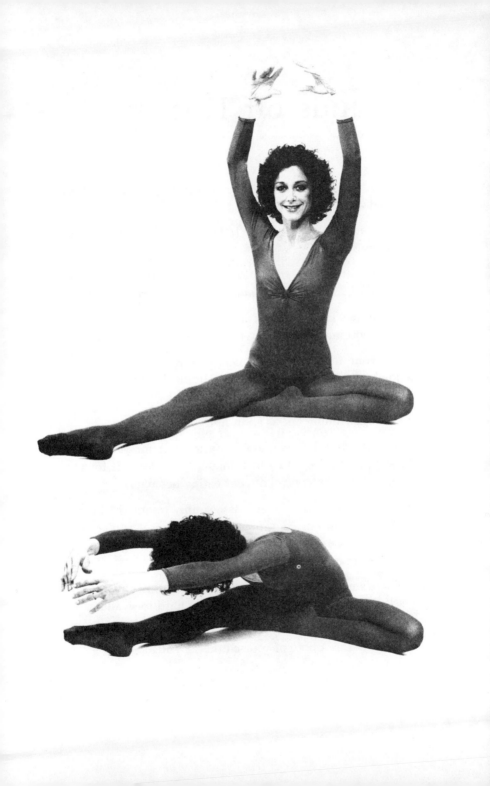

Pounds-off Tips

- Keep active. Boredom leads to eating. Activity relieves boredom.

- Don't eat between meals. It keeps your digestive system overloaded.

- Beware of calorie traps. Purchase a good pocket calorie counter and keep it on hand for occasional referral.

- Make an "event" out of a meal. Set an attractive table, play soothing music, be creative in your food preparation.

- Put your fork and spoon down between mouthfuls. Eat slowly. It takes at least twenty minutes for the stomach to signal the brain that it is satisfied.

- Don't use dining out as an excuse to overeat.

- Lose weight when you are ready to do it for *yourself,* not for someone else. Only by thinking "I'm doing it for me," can you stay in control of your eating behavior.

- If you go off your diet one day, simply resume it the next. Don't throw in the towel just because you've been naughty. Remember, you're only human. Forgive, forget, and forge on!

- There's no avoiding it, a successful diet must involve some self-denial, though the fact might be hard to swallow. You must eat *less.*

- Paste a "fat" photo of yourself on the fridge.

Week III
Introduction

It takes lots of discipline and dedication to stick to a daily at-home exercise program. There's always the temptation to place exercise on a "back burner" and do something else. Never consider it a luxury that you might "squeeze" into your busy day. You probably won't. Instead, make it a daily habit. Your sessions should be an important and necessary part of your beauty regimen—like applying your makeup or taking a bath. Place it high on your list of priorities. And if you find your enthusiasm growing sluggish, remind yourself that the payoff in both mental and physical terms is well worth the effort.

1. Twister

Placement: Sit tall with your legs extended as far to the sides as possible, toes pointed. Rest your hands on your legs.

Movement: Twist your upper body to the left. Lower your torso and head over the leg. Reach for the foot with your right hand. Gently bounce up and down five times. Lift to the beginning position, then repeat to the right.

Repetition: Repeat six times on each side.

As you reach for your foot, keep your buttock as stationary as possible and your head relaxed. Each time you return to center position, don't forget to sit tall.

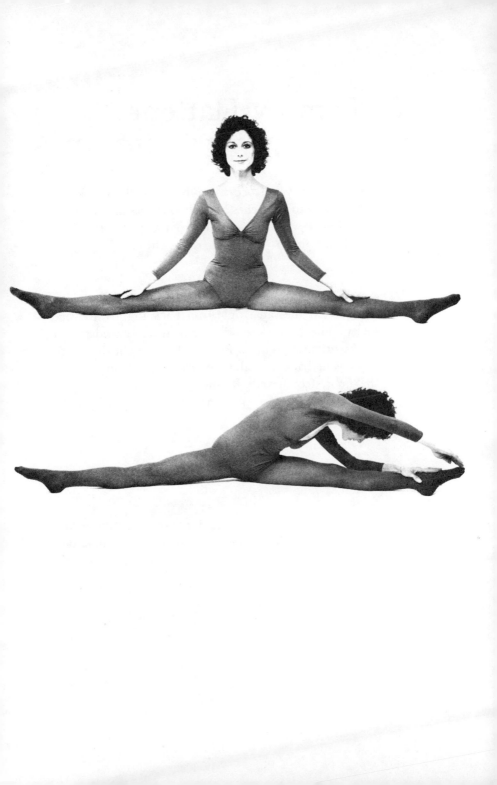

2. Tummy Flattener

Placement: Sit on your coccyx (tailbone) with your knees drawn close to your chest. Point your toes and position the soles of your feet parallel to the floor. Interlace your hands under your knees, elbows lifted.

Movement: Extend both legs forward until they are straight. At the same time, roll back slightly to your lower spine as you extend your arms to the sides. Lift to the original position. Repeat slowly eight times. To relax your back and abdominals, extend your legs on the floor, feet flexed. Round your back, lower your head, and reach for your toes. Bounce up and down eight times.

Repetition: Repeat the sequence four times.

Exhale as you extend your legs forward. The more you contract your abdominals, the easier it will be to maintain balance and control. This is a tricky exercise; give yourself time to perfect it.

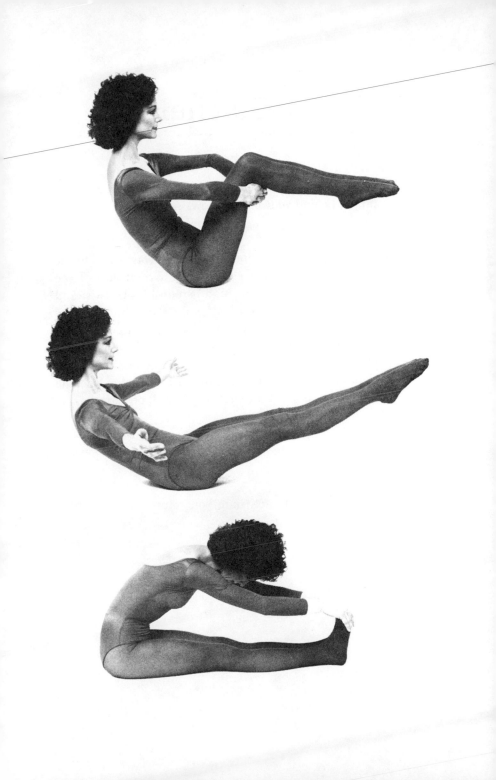

3. Waist Cincher

Placement: Sit tailor fashion, back erect. Interlace your fingers behind your head, elbows wide apart.

Movement: Twist your upper body from your waist to the right. Lower your left elbow to your right knee. Keep the right elbow lifted as high as possible. Untwist and lift to the original position, pulling up through your torso. Repeat to the left. Repeat eight times to each side. Relax by rounding your back, lowering your head, and bringing your elbows together. Hold for eight counts, then uncurl vertebra by vertebra opening the elbows as you lift to a straight-back position.

Repetition: Repeat the sequence three times.

Remember to sit tall each time you return to center position.

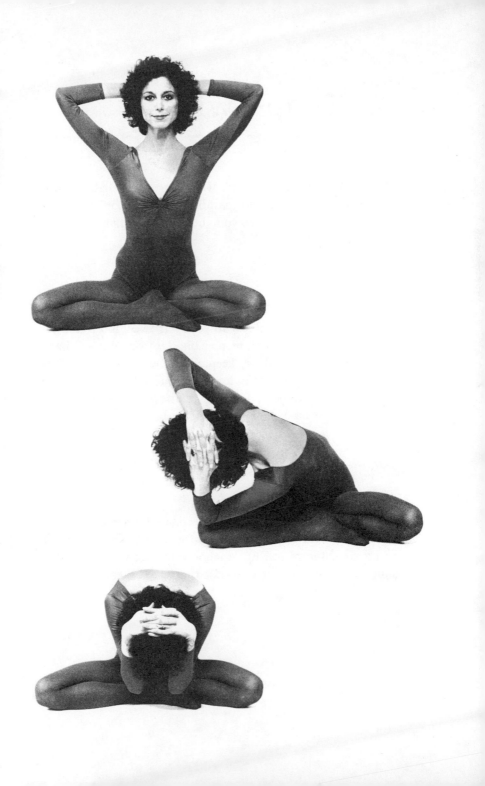

4. Sit-up Twist

Placement: Lie on your back with your knees slightly bent, feet wide apart and parallel on the floor. Interlace your fingers and rest your head in your hands, elbows touching the floor.

Movement: Contract your abdominals. Slowly roll up off the floor and twist your upper body to the left. Try to touch your right elbow to your left knee. Keep the left elbow raised as high as possible. Untwist and roll back down onto the floor, keeping the elbows pointed forward and your chin low. Let the elbows touch the floor last. Repeat, twisting to the right. Repeat four times to each side. Rest for eight slow counts.

Repetition: Repeat this sequence three times.

As you roll back to the floor, vertebra by vertebra, keep your abdominal and buttock muscles tightly contracted. If you are unable to roll up, anchor your feet under a stable support and practice the exercise that way instead.

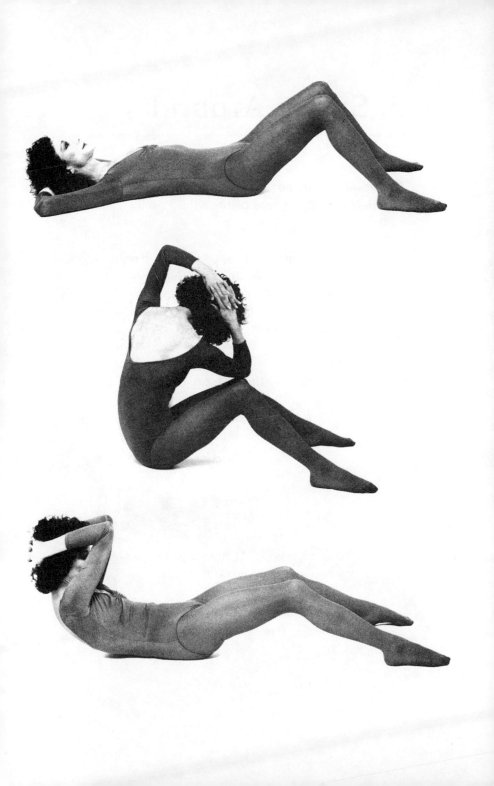

5. Swing Around

Placement: Begin on your hands and knees. Extend the right leg behind, toes pointed.

Movement: Keeping the toes pointed and resting on the floor, swing the leg as far to the right then as far to the left as possible. Follow the movement of your leg with your head. Repeat the total swing eight times. Then repeat with the left leg.

Repetition: Repeat two times on each leg.

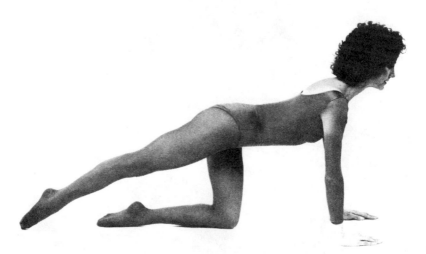

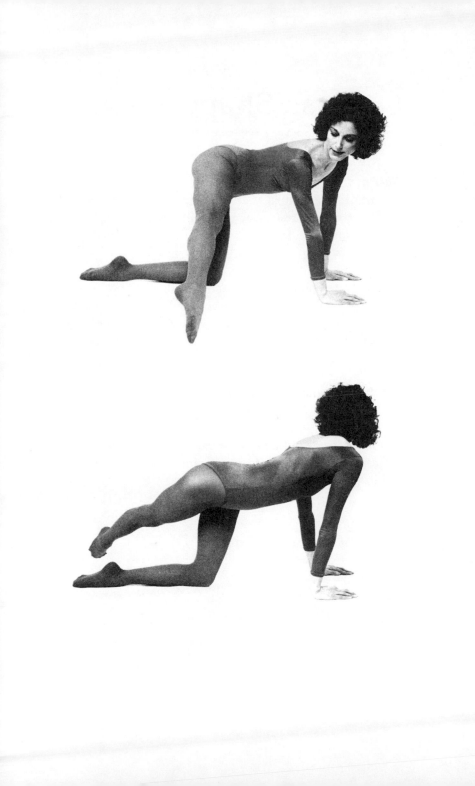

6. Torso Shaper

Placement: Lie on your back with your legs extended toward the ceiling, knees slightly bent. Interlace your fingers and rest your head in your hands, elbows touching the floor.

Movement: Contract your abdominals. Lift your head, neck, and shoulders off the floor as you bring your elbows close to your knees. Repeat eight times. Next, draw your knees to your chest and hold for six counts.

Repetition: Repeat the sequence three times.

You absolutely must work on a padded surface for this exercise, so as not to bruise your spine. Each time you lift, pull in your abdominals and exhale.

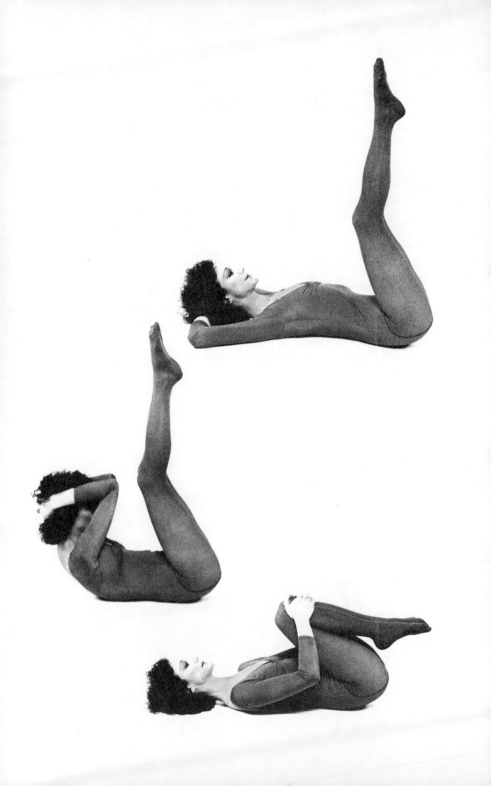

7. Side Bounce

Placement: Sit with your right leg extended to the side, toes pointed. Bend your left leg and place the foot close to your body. Keep your shoulders in line with your hips.

Movement: Lean and stretch your upper body to the right. Reach for your right foot with your right hand as your left arm arches overhead, palm up. Bounce up and down four times. Return to the original position. Repeat six times. Then repeat to the left.

Repetition: Repeat two times on each side.

Keep your buttocks stationary as you stretch to the side.

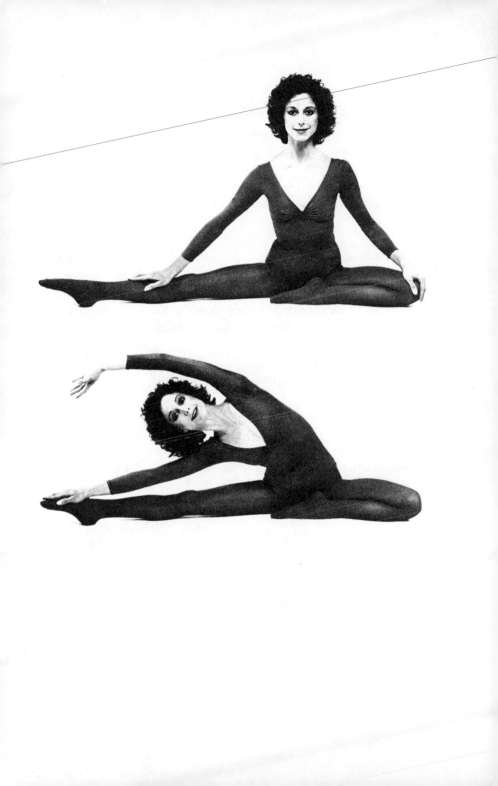

8. Calf Grasp

Placement: Lie on your back, legs extended in front, toes pointed. Rest your arms on the floor overhead.

Movement: Lift your right leg as high as possible. At the same time swing your arms and upper body forward, clasping your hands around your leg near the calf. Hold for four counts, then slowly roll back to the floor, arms stretched overhead. Repeat with the left leg.

Repetition: Repeat eight times on each leg.

Before lifting, contract and take a full exhalation. Try not to lift too high. Stop at your maximum stress point so that you are supported by your lower spine. In order for this exercise to be somewhat less difficult, you may bend the extended leg and place the foot on the floor.

Running in Place

(Three minutes)

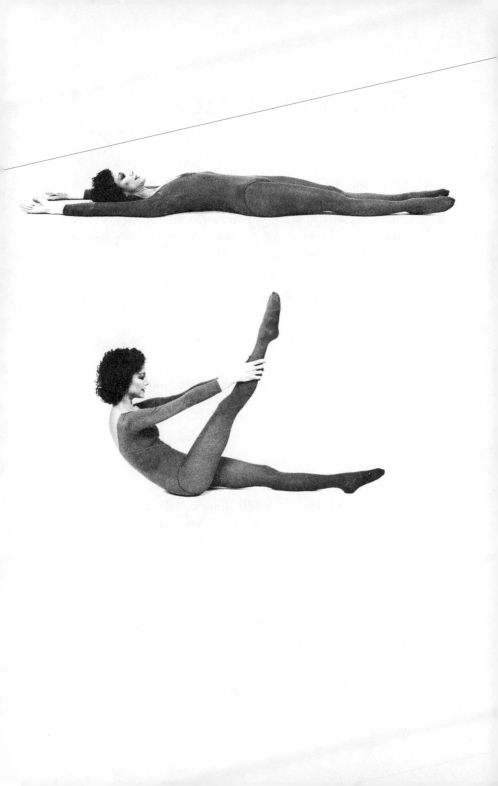

Slim-down Tips

- Separate the idea of character building from the idea of losing weight. Instead of constantly putting willpower to the test, start to work out strategies so you won't have to test your willpower all the time. Who says it's wrong to make things easier for yourself?

- Take up something new . . . a hobby or interest. It helps take your mind off eating, and it occupies your hands which otherwise put food into your mouth.

- Don't skip meals. Instead, cut out the in-between "munching" that really puts on the pounds.

- Make a list of situations in which you find that you overeat: for example, watching television, reading, at parties, when you're upset. Put the list in a prominent place and add to it as new situations confront you.

- Change your daily routine in order to make it more exercise and action packed.

- Be aware of how often you think or talk about food, then start focusing on other things. If you continue to focus on recipes, eating, and how fat you feel and look, you're still too involved with food.

- Ask yourself if you really want what you're about to eat. Oftentimes, the answer will be no, and you will have saved considerable calories in the asking.

- Drink a glass of water before each meal. It's filling.

- Don't skip breakfast. It need not be a huge meal, but do eat something nutritious to get your day started right.

Week IV
Introduction

You've come a long way baby . . . but the exercises in this
week's segment are the most demanding thus far. It might
take a day or so, perhaps even more, to feel comfortable
with all eight exercises. Don't push yourself beyond capac-
ity. Take one day at a time and work toward perfecting the
movements. Above all, stay with it, no matter how busy
you might be. Commitment is the key! In fact, the busier
you are and the more responsibilities you assume, the more
crucial it is that you feel and look your best. Keep it up
. . . you're doing great!

1. Kick Back

Placement: Begin on your hands and knees with your hands shoulder-width apart. Bend your right knee toward your chest, back rounded, chin low.

Movement: Swing the leg back and up as you lift your torso and head. Repeat rhythmically eight times. Repeat with the left leg.

Repetition: Repeat three times with each leg.

Exhale and contract your abdominals each time you round your back.

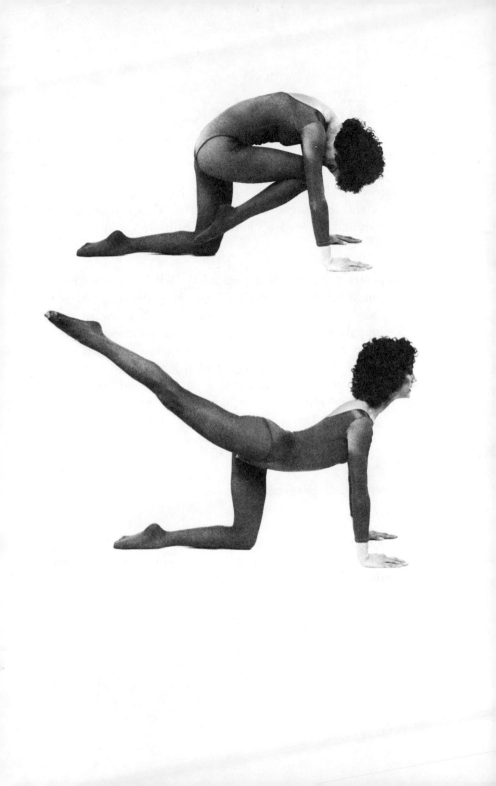

2. Flutter Kick

Placement: Lie on your back, left leg extended upward, right leg extended on the floor. Clasp your hands around the left leg, close to the calf.

Movement: Release your grip on the left leg and lower it until the foot is practically touching the floor. At the same time raise your right leg and pull it toward you, hands near the calf. Change hands rhythmically from one leg to the other as you pull each leg toward your body. Repeat six times on each leg. Then repeat the same movement, this time with your head, neck, and shoulders lifted off the floor. Repeat six times on each leg. To relax your neck, lower your head, draw your knees to your chest and rest six slow counts.

Repetition: Repeat the entire sequence four times.

As you change legs, try to keep them as straight as possible, toes pointed. Hold your abdominals in and keep your breathing steady.

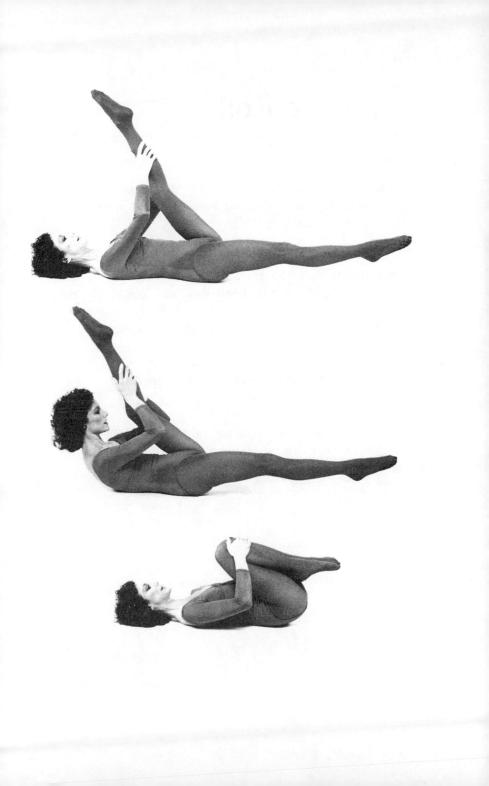

3. Knee Roll

Placement: Lie on your back with your knees drawn close to your chest. Rest your hands on your waist, elbows touching the floor.

Movement: Roll your knees to the left. Extend both legs to the left, diagonally. Bend them and roll to the right. Repeat six times to each side. Rest by drawing your knees to your chest and holding for six counts.

Repetition: Repeat the sequence three times.

As you roll your knees to the sides, keep them together. Exhale as you extend the legs, inhale as you roll.

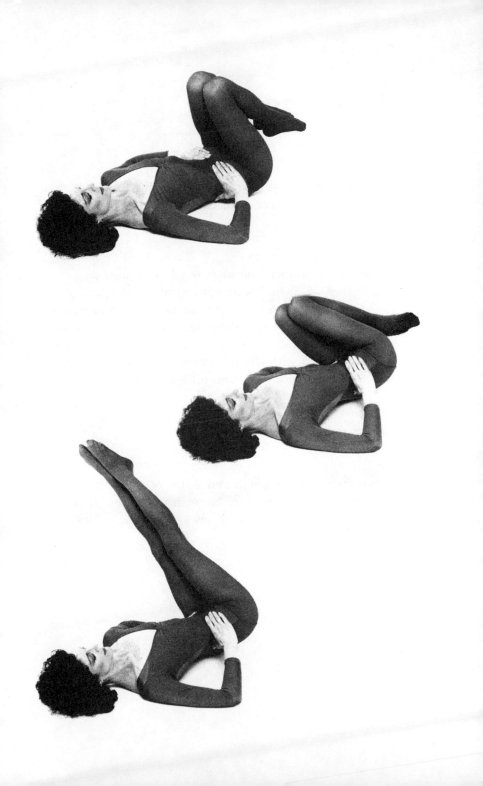

4. Swing Up

Placement: Lie on your back, legs extended in front, toes pointed. Rest your arms on the floor overhead, palms up.

Movement: Contract your abdominals and press your back against the floor. Swing your arms up and forward as you simultaneously lift your upper body and legs off the floor. Try to grasp your legs near the calf and support yourself on your tailbone. Hold for three counts. Slowly and with control, lower your legs and body to the original position, arms releasing overhead.

Repetition: Repeat twelve times.

This exercise is quite tough and will take some practice before you feel totally comfortable with it. Make certain you lower your body and legs as slowly as possible.

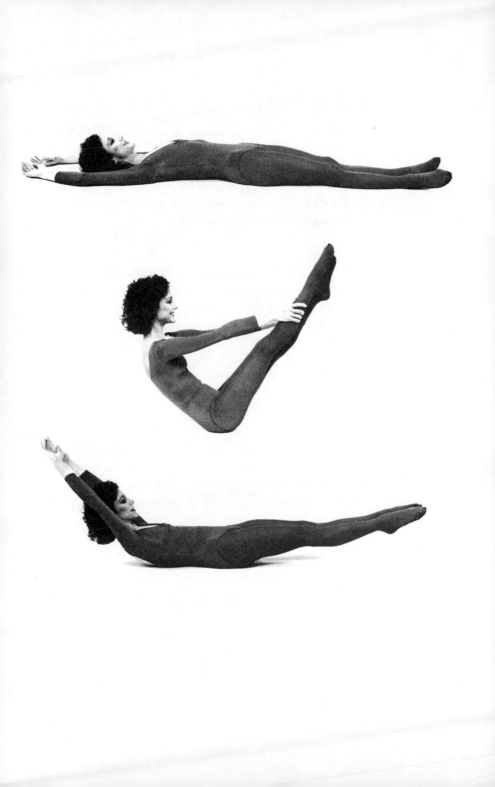

5. Leg Lift

Placement: Lie on your right side. Use your right elbow and left hand to support your torso, which should be raised. Lift your left leg as high as possible.

Movement: Lift the right leg and try to bring the foot in front of the left foot. Lower the leg, then lift it again and try to bring the foot behind the left foot. Repeat this two-part leg lift six times. Roll over and repeat on the left side.

Repetition: Repeat three times on each side.

If you are unable to keep the upper leg raised without support, clasp your hand around it in order to maintain the lift. Keep your waist off the floor and your upper body facing forward as much as possible. Exhale each time you raise the leg.

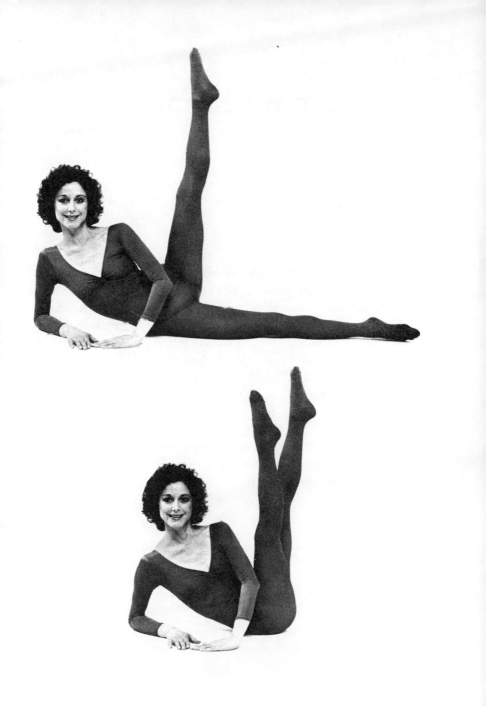

6. Tummy Firmer

Placement: Lie on your back with your legs extended up, toes pointed. Rest your arms on the floor overhead.

Movement: Swing your arms up and forward as you lift your head, neck, shoulders, and upper back off the floor. Try to touch your hands to your legs. Release to the original position. Repeat eight times, then relax with your legs extended on the floor, gently rolling your head from side to side six times.

Repetition: Repeat the sequence three times.

As you lift off the floor, exhale and contract your abdominals. Make certain to lower your chin so as not to place unnecessary strain on your neck.

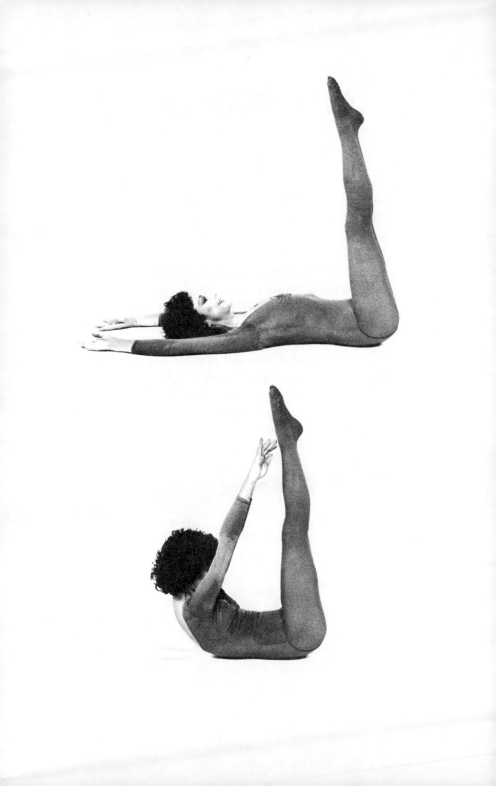

7. Waist Whittler

Placement: Sit with your legs extended out to the sides, toes pointed. Interlace your fingers and place your hands behind your head, elbows open to the sides.

Movement: Twist your upper body from the waist to your right. Keep your elbows wide apart. Lower your torso over your leg, trying to touch your left elbow to your right knee. Keep your right elbow lifted. Raise your torso and return to center position, then twist to your left. Repeat six times to each side. Next, to relax your back, lower your head, round your back, and bring your elbows together. Bounce up and down six times. Uncurl slowly until you resume the original straight-back position.

Repetition: Repeat the sequence three times.

Try to keep your upper elbow raised as you lower your body.

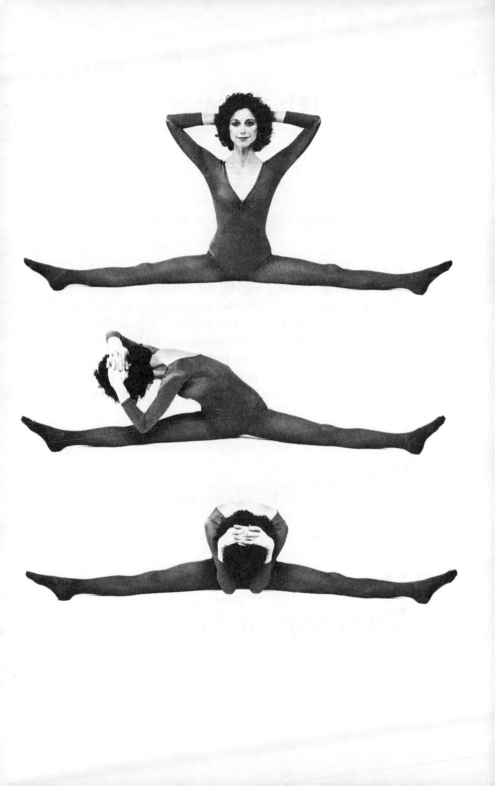

8. Waist-away

Placement: Lie on your back with your knees bent close to your chest. Interlace your fingers and rest your head in your hands, elbows touching the floor.

Movement: Extend your right leg forward until it is straight and raised slightly off the floor, toes pointed. At the same time, lift your head, neck, and shoulders and try to touch your right elbow to your left knee. Next, bend the right leg, straighten the left, and try to touch the left elbow to the right knee. Repeat three times on each leg. Then draw your knees to your chest and gently roll your head from side to side six times.

Repetition: Repeat the sequence three times.

When extending the leg forward, keep it as close to the floor as possible. If you wish to take a longer pause to relax your neck, take several more counts.

Running in Place

(Three minutes)

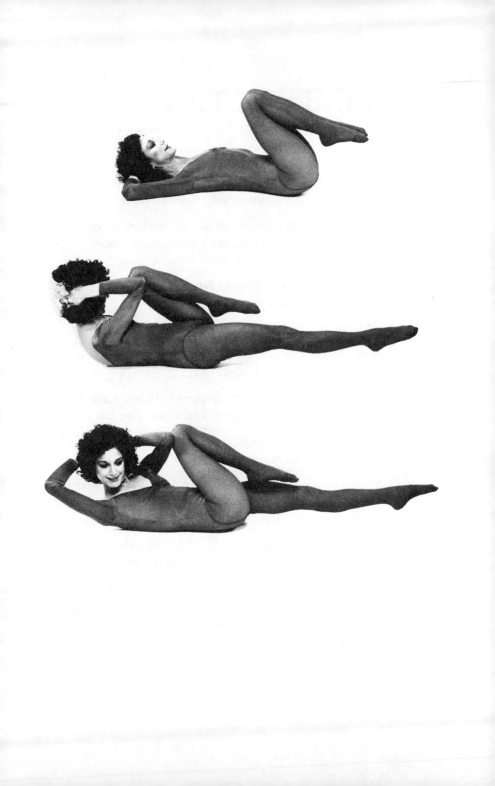

Trim-down Tips

- Celebrate your weight loss with a non-food treat . . . a pedicure, a bunch of daisies, your favorite perfume.

- If you can't resist the temptation of certain foods once you've brought them home, don't bring them home in the first place.

- Remember, the "tastes" you devour while cooking and the leftovers you finish do count.

- Don't let others sabotage your diet.

- Beware of diet plateaus. You're bound to hit a period when the pounds won't budge. Don't give up!

- You don't have to "clean your plate." Leave some food. Better to *waste* it than to have it appear on your *waist*.

- A glass of grapefruit juice is a convenient midday pick-me-up and ideal for staving off hunger pangs.

- Don't skip meals the day of a dinner party. Going without breakfast and lunch won't save calories at all if you end up being so starved that you gorge on anything in sight.

- At a buffet party, scout the table from end to end *before* you make your selections. Once you know what foods are available, you can choose wisely.

- Weight control is as simple as ABC: Step up your *AC-TIVITY*. Take note of your eating *BEHAVIOR*. Decrease your *CALORIES*.

A Final Note. . .

I hope this book has motivated and inspired you to make exercise part of your daily beauty regimen. If you've made the commitment, you've taken the most important step toward a future of lasting good looks, poise, and vitality.

You've worked hard and diligently to achieve your figure goals—a slimmer waist and trimmer tummy. Congratulations! Now, perhaps, you might wish to devote time to firming and toning other problem zones (if you have them). You'll find a terrific collection of easy-to-follow, effective spot toners in my book, *Barbara Pearlman's Slendercises.* Or, if you prefer a head-to-toe fifteen-minute-a-day program, my book, *Barbara Pearlman's Dance Exercises* is the ideal eight-week plan for you.

Your personal, at-home exercise program should be a lifelong, long-life activity. By adopting the "exercise habit," a lovely figure and lively health are yours to have, not for a week or a month, but for the rest of your life.